IN THE
NATIONAL INTEREST

General Sir John Monash once exhorted a graduating class to 'equip yourself for life, not solely for your own benefit but for the benefit of the whole community'. At the university established in his name, we repeat this statement to our own graduating classes, to acknowledge how important it is that common or public good flows from education.

Universities spread and build on the knowledge they acquire through scholarship in many ways, well beyond the transmission of this learning through their education. It is a necessary part of a university's role to debate its findings, not only with other researchers and scholars, but also with the broader community in which it resides.

Publishing for the benefit of society is an important part of a university's commitment to free intellectual inquiry. A university provides civil space for such inquiry by its scholars, as well as for investigations by public intellectuals and expert practitioners.

This series, In the National Interest, embodies Monash University's mission to extend knowledge and encourage informed debate about matters of great significance to Australia's future.

Professor Margaret Gardner AC
President and Vice-Chancellor,
Monash University

BILL BOWTELL
UNMASKED: THE POLITICS OF PANDEMICS

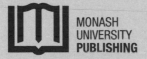

MONASH
UNIVERSITY
PUBLISHING

Monash University Publishing
Matheson Library Annexe
40 Exhibition Walk
Monash University
Clayton, Victoria 3800, Australia
https://publishing.monash.edu

Monash University Publishing brings to the world publications which advance the best traditions of humane and enlightened thought.

ISBN: 9781922464248 (paperback)
ISBN: 9781922464262 (ebook)

Series: In the National Interest
Editor: Louise Adler
Project manager & copyeditor: Paul Smitz
Designer: Peter Long
Typesetter: Cannon Typesetting
Proofreader: Gillian Armitage
Printed in Australia by Ligare Book Printers

A catalogue record for this book is available from the National Library of Australia.

The paper this book is printed on is in accordance with the standards of the Forest Stewardship Council®. The FSC® promotes environmentally responsible, socially beneficial and economically viable management of the world's forests.

PREFACE

In this book, I draw on four decades' experience at and around the intersection of politics and pandemics. This stretches from how Australia and the world responded to HIV/AIDS in the 1980s to the grim circus of coronavirus and COVID-19 in 2020.

I survived the mayhem and carnage of HIV/AIDS. I saw at close quarters how cynical politicians and poor decisions led directly to millions of deaths, severe and avoidable illnesses, and social upheaval. I did not think that this could happen again. But I was mistaken.

We must understand both what went so wrong and what was done well. We should learn from those who did better. And we must discard those structures and assumptions that served us poorly, replacing them with structures and policies that in the future will better anticipate, contain, manage and eliminate viral challenges with the least possible toll of injury, death, and economic and social disruption.

Above all, it is imperative that we strengthen our own public health infrastructure and the international public health architecture centred on the World Health Organization (WHO) and other agencies.

And we have to do this now. We can never know when the next viral threat will come along, only that it is inevitable and can happen anytime and anywhere.

I am Australian and my views are drawn predominantly though not exclusively from my career in Australian public life. The narrative here around the emergence of coronavirus is set in the context of how things developed in Australia over 2020.

Australia is a geographically large country with a relatively small population. It is governed by a complex federal edifice created in 1901 that melded together the models of Washington and Westminster. This might have been the height of enlightened nineteenth-century liberal political thinking, but, like its parents in the United Kingdom and the United States, Australia's federation has far outlived its usefulness. It has become a dead weight around the neck of Australia's democracy and people. Our ramshackle government structures are outmoded and cannot cope with the scope and gravity of the planetary emergencies that confront us.

We are a complex and sophisticated country now greatly hobbled by simplistic and unsophisticated politics and politicians. The ease with which a simple virus inflicted serious, lasting damage on the health, wealth and happiness of the Australian people is the clearest possible evidence that things have gone badly wrong. The levers of democratic power have moved from the people to a very few whose visions and instincts are no longer grounded in building 'common wealth', and who cannot be trusted to act in the national rather than sectional interest. The fractured response to coronavirus is just the latest in a long list of policy failures that have diminished the nation's capacity to deal with the foreseeable problems and challenges hurtling towards us.

It appears that we are about at the end of the beginning of the pandemic, with much more to endure before better times return. So while it is still too early to write a comprehensive history of how and why things turned out so badly, we have been through enough for me to make a start.

In writing this book, I have done my best to base my conclusions and views on a fair assessment of the facts and evidence as disclosed on the public record. But I have been greatly hampered by the fact that all the documents, minutes, proceedings and even the memberships of the key advisory committees have been declared state secrets.[1] Lacking access to these records, I have relied on public interviews, articles, and many informal and illuminating discussions with senior politicians, officials and front-line personnel at every level.

On 8 April 2020, the Australian Senate established the Select Committee on COVID-19, chaired by Senator Katy Gallagher.[2] The committee is doing sterling work in attempting to hold Australian ministers and officials to account. I have also drawn on evidence given to the select committee and the various other committees established to investigate and report on the significant events and lapses in the administration of Australia's pandemic experience.

Many opinions and views have been shared on social media. Assertions without evidence are just that and should always be discounted. But I have found there are many thoughtful and incisive interlocutors on social media who have timely, evidence-based insights. If journalism is the first draft of history, then Twitter has become, for better or worse, the first draft of journalism.

It may be that consulting the secret and confidential records held by the governments of Australia will lead me to revise some of my conclusions, or to recast the actions of some of those involved in making coronavirus policy in a more favourable light. As and when the truth is disclosed to the Australian people, I will of course be delighted to correct any errors of fact or judgement.

This book will be published in early 2021, some months after it was written. If, when it appears, Australia has maintained zero local transmissions and thereby avoided a national second wave, and if Victoria has avoided a third wave, that will be entirely due to the good sense of the Australian people in implementing policies based on science, not politics. Anything short of that will be the result of politics trumping science.

Bill Bowtell AO
Sydney, October 2020

UNMASKED: THE POLITICS OF PANDEMICS

Nature creates viruses. But politics creates pandemics. And pandemics create new politics.

Politics is process. It is as essential to human development as viruses are to evolution. Politics is how human beings build societies, by arguing and agreeing, more or less, about how resources are to be divided and to what purpose. Politics reflects and shapes the human condition.

But it is inherently and always conditional, relative, improvised, incomplete, an expression of whim, fashion and frenzy. As a process involving fallible human beings, it can never deliver absolute truths about human affairs. There are no 'iron laws' of politics, or society or economics, just as there can never be iron laws of culture, music, arts, literature or beauty.

Yet in every generation over the centuries, humans seeking wealth and power over others claim to have discovered just those immutable, transcendent iron laws, truths and principles which, if applied, will bring order to the chaos of human life. These fabricators of stories and myth play on the insatiable human desire for hope, an end to the endless journey, for peace and quiet in this world or the next. By claiming to explain the universe, they lead their followers to believe that the universe is also controllable by them.

But they are wrong. Politics and science have never mixed well. Science is grounded in the belief that the reality of the universe is objectively so, and that it exists without human agency, permission or politics.

Science has provided staggeringly powerful tools that have transformed the world and destroyed and created empires and societies. And politicians have always sought to harness and subordinate the insights of science in the pursuit of their political goals and objectives. But the problem is that the truths of politics and science cannot both be right. Either truth is relative and shaped politically, or it is absolute and objectively so, beyond any ability of humans to alter or deny that reality.

There are indeed iron laws that govern and explain all things. But these are not the laws of politics. They are instead the laws of physics, chemistry, biology and mathematics.[3]

In 2020, matters have come to a decisive moment in the long struggle between bad politics and science. The world is in the second year of the coronavirus pandemic. The human misery and anguish caused by the virus has been immense. The direct toll of death, illness and infection is in the tens of millions and mounting. Those not directly affected by the virus have suffered from the evaporation of jobs in entire sectors of the global economy and the collapse from growth into recession.

But the carnage was not spread equally among all countries. Some sailed through the emergency phase of the pandemic with low levels of infections and deaths and minimal long-term damage to their economies and societies. Coronavirus remained a serious public health problem but never became more than that. Most, however, failed spectacularly in their efforts to see off the threat of coronavirus, and the problem morphed into a pandemic that up-ended them. How did this happen?

Viruses jump from animals to humans ceaselessly and predictably. They are no more than mindless infection engines whose general characteristics are well understood by science. The properties of coronavirus are the same everywhere. So why did some countries control coronavirus from the outset while many crumbled into its deadly embrace? The difference was entirely down to politics and people.

Those whose leaders saw things for what they were, who planned and prepared and made the right decisions in time to make an impact, came through relatively unscathed. But those whose leaders placed their political interests above public health, science and experience, who hoped for the best while failing to prepare for the worst, turned the problem into a pandemic. In doing so, they visited misery, death and destruction on their people.

Faced with the consequences, these leaders have sought to avoid responsibility and accountability. They proclaim that the emergence of coronavirus was 'unprecedented', 'unpredictable', that its scything progress around the world was 'inevitable', 'unstoppable'. This is rubbish.

The peoples of the world have been badly let down by the venality, mendacity and incompetence of those who failed to stop coronavirus in its tracks or to impede its spread. Prevention is always better and cheaper than cure. The costs of preparing and planning ahead to avoid the worst would have amounted to the tiniest fraction of what the world has been forced to spend to offset the consequences of rampant coronavirus.

In Australia, good luck and geography provided just enough time and space to avert a dumping first wave. Then the commitment and tireless work of tens of thousands of front-line public health workers and officials, combined with the discipline and sacrifice of the Australian people, staved off the worst of the pandemic. But even so, shortcomings in strategy and management caused avoidable infections and deaths, and contributed to the making of policies that have had profoundly bad social and economic impacts.

NATURE CREATES VIRUSES

Viruses are small particles of inanimate matter that replicate by infecting the host cells of living things.

They are an integral part of the natural world. But viruses are not alive. They do not have a cellular structure and cannot reproduce themselves by cellular division. In evolutionary terms, their function is to transmit genes between living organisms. In doing so, viruses perform an essential function for all forms of cellular life, from plants to animals to humans.

Since the beginnings of life on earth, viruses have coexisted in a symbiotic relationship with cellular organisms. Over billions of years, the genetic exchange facilitated by viruses allowed the evolution of life into increasingly complex forms. But as life became more complex, viruses did not. As the number and variety of living things increased, viruses simply colonised them and continued to replicate.

Viruses were here long before us and they will be here long after we are gone. Viruses do not live in our world—we live in theirs. Throughout history, viruses have emerged from nature and infected human beings. They are constantly exchanged between humans and other animals. However, immune systems and viruses are engaged in a perpetual struggle between offence and defence. A virus that is too weak to infect a new host will, of course, disappear. So viruses mutate and evolve. From time to time, a virus evolves characteristics for which the immune system of a prospective animal or human host has no effective blocking response. In such cases, the new virus is able to infect and replicate. In doing so, it can cause immense damage to its unwilling individual host. Successful replication within an infected host greatly increases the chances of the virus transmitting copies of itself to a potential new host. This distribution of genetic material will almost certainly strengthen the capacity of the infected species to evolve. But in the case of human beings, that is very cold comfort to the individual who is sickened, crippled or killed by their encounter with a virus.

Understandably, we are most afraid of a highly infectious viral epidemic emerging without warning and rapidly killing millions before exhausting itself. But from the point of view of the virus, there is such a thing as being too contagious. If too many susceptible hosts perish, or the virus encounters those who are naturally immune to it, it soon reaches the limits of its growth. And fast-acting viruses can be contained by quarantine.

The far more insidious threat to human health arises from what might be called a Goldilocks virus— one that is not too weak, nor too strong, but has just the right characteristics to allow infection and maximum replication, and a long period between first infection and the onset of noticeable symptoms.

Sometimes a new virus fails in its sole purpose of lodging in a new human host and replicating. But overwhelmingly when it comes to encounters between human animals and viruses, viruses prevail.

As the survivors of this or that viral victory over our species survey the carnage, they are often tempted to see in viruses the qualities they most abhor in other human beings. Viruses are described as 'vicious', 'sneaky', 'ruthless' and 'cunning'. Sometimes they are seen as agents of the supernatural, or divine punishment for sin and transgression. Viruses are none of these things. They just are. Becoming emotional about viruses impedes our ability to see things clearly. And by not understanding the true nature of viruses, our collective ability to meet, contain and control their impacts on humanity is diminished rather than strengthened. A clear understanding of the nature of viruses is crucial to their management in human beings.

Prevention is possible only if we understand transmission, the core business of the virus. On the other hand, prevention is the business of humans. Prevention is political. The transmission and spread of any viral infection can, in theory, be controlled and contained. Highly infectious human carriers can be isolated or quarantined. All we need to know to control the spread of a new virus is where it lies on the scale of contagiousness and what human practices are implicated in its transmission.

The initial response must of course be grounded in well-established public health protocols that respond to the contagious and infectious properties of the new virus. In time, scientific investigation and research will almost certainly deliver reasonably effective therapies and treatments, and possibly vaccines or cures.

The social and political challenge is to persuade or oblige people to change behaviours for as long as it takes until the development of useful treatments or vaccines.

Over the centuries, armed with ever-increasing knowledge, the world has become better able to cope with the emergence of viruses. Still, the difference between success and failure has always been a function of the political response to the virus.

One of the greatest achievements of public health in the late twentieth century was the successful eradication of smallpox. By the end of World War II, smallpox had been brought under control and virtually eliminated in the developed countries. However, the disease was still killing millions of people in the developing countries. In 1959 alone, fifty million people were infected with smallpox and over two million people died. Led by the WHO, a global program to eliminate smallpox began in 1958 and was intensified in 1967. Concentrated vaccination campaigns, complemented by the quarantining of outbreaks, were undertaken region by region. On 9 December 1979, a committee of eminent scientists confirmed the eradication of smallpox, and this was endorsed by the World Health Assembly on 8 May 1980. It was a triumph of the application of public health principles and methods.

But the greatest achievement of international public health and global cooperation was being proclaimed and celebrated just as the HIV virus began its deadly progress from Africa to the rest of the world. In virology, nemesis is sure to follow hubris.

POLITICS CREATES PANDEMICS

The human immunodeficiency virus (HIV) originated decades if not centuries ago in central African primates. The earliest known human case detected by blood sample dates from 1959. Thanks to its stealthy characteristics, HIV spread undetected in rural and remote Africa for decades, moving slowly and, for a long time, imperceptibly in bodily fluids exchanged relatively infrequently. Onset of the symptoms of acquired immune deficiency syndrome (AIDS) followed many months or years after HIV infection. Its slow-acting, long-lasting nature made it much harder to identify, contain, manage and prevent than, for example, an influenza virus. Whenever semen or blood was exchanged, there was a route for transmission of the still-undetected virus.

Sometime in the 1970s, HIV crossed the Atlantic. The HIV epidemic had already claimed many African lives, but its prehistory counted for nothing when it finally hit America. In 1981, the 'first' case of HIV/AIDS infection was noticed in New York City among sexually active gay men, and the politicisation of the syndrome transformed a problem into a pandemic. The emergence of AIDS within Manhattan's highly sexually active gay community was simply a random, chance event. But the timing and nature of this first appearance in America had catastrophic consequences for the subsequent course of events, both in the United States and globally.

Almost immediately after the disease was first reported, the debate about its nature, causes and possible treatment became hopelessly enmeshed in the toxic stew of American domestic politics. The political struggle between secular liberalism and a resurgent fundamentalist Christianity had been simmering since the 1960s and erupted with great force following Ronald Reagan's election as president in 1980. AIDS became a cause and symbol to both sides of the American culture wars. America rebranded, repositioned and repackaged the syndrome for the world. It became the 'gay plague', the 'wages of sin' as foretold in Biblical prophecy. (Four decades later, the 'paranoid style' in American politics was reprised in conjuring up explanations for the emergence of coronavirus.)[4]

Throughout the 1980s, America's political leaders ignored or discounted the emerging body of scientific evidence about the nature of AIDS. Moves towards a rational and measured response were repeatedly swamped by the forces of religious reaction, which were determined to associate the disease with the sinful trinity of homosexuality, prostitution and drugs. Effective prevention required official recognition of sexual activity and diversity, and illicit drug use. Yet the Reagan administration, the national government of the richest, most diverse nation in the world, took no swift, effective measures at a time when it almost certainly could have stalled the spread of HIV.

The politicisation of AIDS in the United States had global consequences, just as the politicisation of coronavirus has four decades later.

SCIENCE, EVIDENCE AND FACT

The first Australian case of HIV was reported in Sydney just a few months before the election in March 1983 of the Hawke Labor government, which had to deal with this mystery ailment from its first weeks in office. After the election, the new health minister, Dr Neal Blewett, appointed me as his senior private secretary—in contemporary terms, his chief of staff. As senior adviser to the health minister, I became a focal point for everyone with an opinion about the dramatic emergence of this exotic disease.

Public concern rose as increasing numbers of cases were reported among gay men in major Australian cities. Contrary to the advice of the Department of Health, the new government was not prepared to leave the matter with the state and territory governments and avoid responsibility for taking whatever steps might need to be taken to respond to the problem. Dr Blewett decided that the federal government would assume national responsibility for handling what soon became a serious emergency and threat to public health. At the time, we had no idea how far and fast this assumption of responsibility would lead us along the path of radical policy innovation.

By 1984 the viral nature of the illness had been identified and a test was developed. HIV was found in bodily fluids but it only seemed to be transmissible in the exchange of blood and semen—though, even then, not always. In the meantime, two schools of thought had developed. The first, shaped by the American debate, pressed for highly repressive measures—sanction, isolation, punishment and quarantine—to be directed at the groups at greatest risk of infection: gay men, sex workers and injecting drug users.

The other school included those closest to the problem: doctors, nurses and those caring for HIV-infected people; clinical scientists researching the virus; bureaucrats involved in the response; secular and religious social workers supporting various at-risk communities; and, most importantly, those with the disease or at risk of contracting it. The emerging scientific evidence showed that the virus was not overly contagious, and our discussions with at-risk groups indicated that they comprised responsible citizens willing and able to educate their peers about moderating risky behaviours. This school acknowledged that what was required was a national strategy to prevent, not accept, transmission of HIV.

Policies had to be based on science, evidence and fact. And remarkably, at the most senior levels of the

Australian Government and parliament, there was almost complete acceptance of this principle: effective policies needed to be funded and applied, and technologies provided, to allow people to protect themselves and their partners from possible infection. Minimising the risk of sexual transmission required the widespread promotion and distribution of condoms. Further, minimising the risk of blood-borne infection required the routine testing of the blood supply for transfusions, and the provision of sterile needles and syringes to people who injected drugs.

In April 1987, the Australian Government opted to support a radical package of HIV-prevention measures. The package was approved by all the political parties represented in the federal parliament. This put Australia's response to HIV/AIDS on a secure, long-term political foundation. These policies comprised timely, peer-based, direct and explicit preventive education campaigns directed both at high-risk groups and the general public; the widespread introduction of subsidised needle and syringe programs, and rapid expansion of methadone maintenance treatment; access to free, anonymous and universal HIV testing; subsidised access to antiretroviral treatments; general advocacy of the need to adopt safer sexual practices, especially the use of condoms; and the widespread availability of condoms and targeted safe-sex messages.

These policies were in turn based on long-term thinking; the primacy of empirical research and evidence in making policy; the need to minimise the risk to the general population; recognition of the importance of research, especially epidemiology, clinical treatment, retrovirology and social science; respect for human rights, to be buttressed as required by legislation; and collaboration and partnership between all those with a stake in the fight.

Major public education and information campaigns alerted Australians to the threat posed by HIV and told them how to prevent infection. Access to clean needles and syringes quickly reduced the worrying rise in infections among injecting drug users. The rates of testing and condom use increased dramatically. Knowledge of the disease, and the facts about its nature and transmission, improved considerably. Over time, incidents of discrimination against HIV-positive people decreased as ignorance and fear declined. The necessary financial and human resources were put behind a clear and unambiguous strategy.

From 1987, the rates of new infection, which had already started to come down in gay men, fell rapidly. The availability of excellent treatments dramatically changed the outlook for the path and nature of HIV infection in Australia and globally. Australia had acted decisively and comprehensively and was rewarded with a much lower overall toll of infection and death than other countries.

The policies funded by the Australian Government in 1987 were those which, on the evidence, were already working best to contain the problem, or which offered a reasonable chance of success in the future. As each intervention was tried, the results were measured, analysed and reported. This was the classical application of the scientific method as the basis for policymaking. We relied most for advice on those closest to the problem. We created advisory structures that encouraged bold and innovative proposals without being compromised by bureaucratic timidity and naysaying. And these proposals were then funded and implemented in the shortest possible time, with the greatest possible impact.

The qualities of the virus were no different in Australia than elsewhere. The difference was the political will to inform, educate, and provide the necessary simple technologies: condoms and clean needles.

THE VIRUS ISN'T THE PROBLEM

The HIV crisis need never have happened. There is nothing inherent in the virus that made inevitable its transition from serious problem to pandemic. The truth is that the major driver of the global spread of HIV was the lack of political will to translate scientific evidence into effective containment policies. The catastrophe of the global HIV/AIDS pandemic was almost entirely the result of a failure to act on the basis of the compelling evidence that was put before responsible policymakers.

When HIV/AIDS emerged in the early 1980s, Australia quickly saw the dreadful mistakes being made in the United States and elsewhere. We turned to our own experts and the most affected communities to craft an Australian response that, over time, came to be seen as among the world's best responses, and which inspired many other countries to do the same.

Our guiding motto was Trust. We told the truth.

From the outset, without panic, we looked to the community to advise, guide and implement the response across care, treatment, research, and above all prevention. We kept nothing secret about modelling, debates, or the ever-improving knowledge we accumulated about the virus, how to avoid infection, and what to do if you acquired it. It never occurred to us to hide anything from the public or the parliament.

Over time, our response—compared with that of the United States of America, for example—saved tens if not hundreds of thousands of Australians from infection with HIV and thousands of Australians from early death from AIDS. And Australia has kept HIV/AIDS under control for almost four decades. The response has been maintained by successive Labor and Liberal–National governments in Canberra and all the states and territories. It has been above and beyond party politics, as these things should be.

The HIV pandemic demonstrated how easy it was for the eruption of a new viral threat to spread from its source to every corner of the globe. It took many years for the world to come to terms with what had to be done to prevent the spread of HIV and to treat all those infected by it. But gradually, sensible policies prevailed and were adopted by most, if not all, countries and regions. By the first decade of the twenty-first century, it seemed that the world had taken to heart the harsh lessons of the failures in the initial response to HIV/AIDS.

From the early 2000s, many other viruses emerged from nature, including severe acute respiratory syndrome (SARS1, in 2002), H1N1 or swine flu (2009), Middle East respiratory syndrome (MERS, 2013), Ebola (2014 and 2018) and Zika (2016). These were all dealt with according to established public health principles implemented under the leadership and direction of the WHO and other agencies. None of these outbreaks were in any way politicised to the point where this impeded or overrode public health goals and the necessary policymaking. In every case, illnesses and deaths were kept to the lowest levels achievable and the outbreaks were contained and eliminated. In most of the developed countries, including Australia, these outbreaks were more or less forgotten as soon as they were contained.

It is easy to see how success engendered complacency. Memories of the failures around HIV receded as those politicians, public health activists, researchers, doctors and philanthropists who built the response faded away. As coronavirus and COVID-19 erupted, the lessons of HIV/AIDS were forgotten. Where there ought to have been trust and openness, there was secrecy. Where public health principles ought to have been applied and policymaking based only on science, evidence and facts, political considerations prevailed. Instead of educating and informing the public, political leaders said that the novel coronavirus threat was 'unprecedented' and 'unpredictable'. What nonsense. From January 2020, what was going to happen was 'precedented' and 'predictable'.

The greatest lesson from HIV/AIDS, and which had to be relearnt when COVID-19 arrived, was this: It's not the virus that's the problem. It's the response.

A NEW VIRAL INFECTION

In late 2019, it took just a few weeks for a submicroscopic particle of non-living matter to shatter the seemingly indestructible foundations of the globalised world. It was able to do so because the greatest emblem of globalisation—the international air transport system—conveyed the virus as rapidly and smoothly around the planet as it did the passengers who were unknowingly carrying the virus in their bodies.

The movement of people and goods is the driver of economic growth and prosperity. It is also a remarkably efficient infection transmission system— especially when international trade is booming and hundreds of millions of people are taking to the skies.

Viruses cannot move of their own accord. The rate at which they spread from one host to another depends on how many infected people travel from place to place. The greater the number of humans that are on the move, the better the chances of a virus replicating, transmitting and surviving.

Four decades of China's great reform had transformed Wuhan, the capital of Hubei province, from a remote provincial city into a major trading hub, seamlessly linked to the globalised world. By 2019, Wuhan Tianhe International Airport had become the fourteenth-busiest airport in China, with almost thirty million passenger journeys per year, and direct international connections to cities and markets in Asia, Europe, North America and Australia. As China became the world's factory, Wuhan prospered from waves of investment in production of all kinds, from heavy industry to consumer goods. The growth of factories and services in and around cities like Wuhan required an immense labour force. This was achieved via a great internal migration from China's rural areas to its cities. In doing so, agricultural workers brought with them their culinary practices, customs and preferences—in particular, their preference for shopping daily for fresh meat, vegetables and fruit. Inevitably, in some places, the standards of market sanitation, animal husbandry and so on failed to keep up with the demands of an expanding population. These were ideal conditions in which a new virus might arise in animals and then infect humans. And once the virus was present in Wuhan's population, the city's excellent transport links offered a rapid way for it to move beyond its place of origin.

In these essential characteristics, Wuhan was no different from countless other cities around the newly globalised world. A new virus will always find a way to evolve and replicate. It is only the questions of where and when a virus will make a successful leap between species that are unknowable and down to random chance. And in late 2019, the ball in this particular game of viral roulette landed in Wuhan.

Perhaps on a farm or in one of the bustling Wuhan markets, a virus evolved in an animal host and began the process of replication. It then transmitted itself from animal to human hosts. The novel virus infected the respiratory tracts of its hosts and generated symptoms that resembled infection by a cold or influenza—runny noses, shortness of breath and shallow coughs, sinus infection and/or headaches. When they were presented with these first cases, Wuhan's doctors could not have known that they were dealing with anything other than the routine symptoms of cold or influenza. However, by late November and early December 2019, some local doctors suspected that they were in fact seeing the emergence of a new viral infection.

On 3 December, Wuhan ophthalmologist Dr Li Wenliang informed a group of fellow doctors that they should protect themselves against infection by an illness that, according to Dr Li's text messages, 'resembled severe acute respiratory syndrome SARS'. After the interception of this message, Dr Li was summoned by local public security authorities and accused of making false statements. To his inestimable credit, Dr Li refused to stay silent as conditions worsened through December. His outspokenness could not help but alert the central government to the existence of a serious problem in Wuhan.[5]

From the public record, it is clear that from early January 2020, China began to make up for the botched initial response by the Wuhan authorities. It began to share crucial knowledge about the emergence, characteristics and spread of coronavirus with the WHO and other agencies and governments, and particularly with the relevant agencies of the US Government. On 11 January, Chinese scientists released the genetic sequence of COVID-19, and on 20 January China confirmed that human-to-human transmission had occurred. Two days later, China sealed off Wuhan and placed its residents into a strict lockdown.

The decision to shut down Wuhan was an all-or-nothing gamble that the spread of the virus beyond the city could be stopped. But just as a virus identifies and overcomes weakness in the body's defences to infect human cells, so too did the new coronavirus exploit the opportunities for spreading inherent in the global air transport system. In the two months between mid-November 2019, when the virus emerged, and 22 January, when Wuhan was sealed off, some 600 000 passengers passed through Wuhan Tianhe International Airport. The closing off of the city, including the cessation of traffic from the airport from 23 January, was the right thing to do to prevent further transmission of the virus within China and around the world. But as sensible as this measure was, it came days if not weeks too late to stop the spread of the virus into the international air transport system.

Over the critical early weeks, there was confusion in China and a marked reluctance by WHO to escalate the emergency and to recommend international travel restrictions. Later in the pandemic, WHO dithered on mask usage and the swift imposition of lockdowns. In mid-2021, the report of the Independent Panel for Pandemic Preparedness and Response, co-chaired by Helen Clark and Ellen Johnson Sirleaf, will give the world a proper understanding of what transpired within China, WHO and internationally in those critical weeks and months from late 2019.[6] But by 1 February, the rest of the world had no rational excuse not to take matters extremely seriously. All the critical information about the nature, infectivity and lethality of the coronavirus threat had been made available by China and confirmed by the WHO, key member states, governments and other agencies. Most significantly, from mid-January, it had been established conclusively that this was a SARS1-type virus and most definitely not a variant of influenza, with all that that meant for pandemic planning. The world now faced a stark set of choices about how to move against coronavirus: 'Let it in' or 'Keep it out'. Should countries where the virus had already entered take heed of China's advice and move decisively to contain outbreaks? And should countries not yet touched by coronavirus infection take every possible measure to stop the virus entering their territories?

Whether they knew it or not, the cities and countries that were geographically closest to China—Taiwan, Vietnam, Hong Kong, Singapore—or most directly linked by high-volume air routes—Italy, the United States—had to decide these matters immediately. The coronavirus had already arrived. Countries that were more remote and had been less affected by coronavirus had somewhat more time.

Any rational assessment of the virological, epidemiological and public health realities could lead to only one conclusion—that in those countries and cities where the virus had taken hold, the most stringent and immediate social-containment measures, perhaps including lockdowns, had to be imposed. In those countries where the virus had not arrived, borders had to be closed, effective surveillance and quarantine measures implemented, and populations placed on high alert and persuaded to make the simple and effective behavioural changes—social distancing, mask-wearing, and hand-washing and other personal hygiene actions—that best impeded transmission.

AMERICA: A FAILURE OF RESPONSIBILITY

It is hard to overstate the critical position that the United States occupies in shaping the global response to public health crises. When the coronavirus emerged, the world should have been able to look to the United States for common sense, measured advice, coordination, support, and the sharing of information about the nature of the threat posed and how best to respond. The US Government knew about coronavirus almost from the moment that it emerged in Wuhan. At first through its own agencies, then through informal advice from Chinese officials, and finally publicly from early January, American public health officials and political leaders knew the outline of the problem, if not initially its full dimensions. It had all the information required to make a tremendous contribution to protecting itself and other countries from the looming pandemic. But it failed in its responsibilities—not just to the American people, but to the world.

When the Trump administration began in 2017, one of its first acts was to disband the national pandemic planning organisation established during the administration of president Obama. Traditionally independent sources of public health advice in the American Government—the Centers for Disease Control and Prevention (CDC), the National Institutes of Health, and the Food and Drug Administration—were relentlessly politicised. President Trump's public statements were initially supportive of China's handling of the virus. However, he was torn between two factions. One wished to politicise the emergence of coronavirus in China as a way of furthering American strategic and economic competition with that nation. The second, 'public health' faction pushed for the administration to take all possible steps to prepare the United States for a coordinated, swift response to coronavirus. Over January 2020, an internal political debate raged between the factions as they tried to reconcile impossibly conflicting demands: what was required to contain the spread of the virus in the United States, and pursuit of the imperatives of politics, trade and economics in the relationship with China. By early February, however, the matter was settled. Political infighting and general chaos resulted in only one thing in terms of public health: American borders were not secured against coronavirus.

President Trump continued to claim publicly that coronavirus posed no threat to the United States. His optimistic assessments were completely at odds with the advice being generated by the CDC, the intelligence community and academic institutions. And the president privately knew the truth, as he confirmed on 7 February in a recorded interview with *Washington Post* associate editor Bob Woodward:

'It goes through air, Bob. That's always tougher than the touch. You know, the touch, you don't have to touch things. Right? But the air, you just breathe the air and that's how it's passed,' he added. 'And so, that's a very tricky one. That's a very delicate one. It's also more deadly than your—you know, your, even your strenuous flus.'[7]

The American people were being falsely reassured that coronavirus was not a serious threat by a president who had been advised differently. But president Trump had an explanation for his caution. 'Well, I think, Bob, really, to be honest with you … I wanted to always play it down,' he told Woodward on 19 March.[8]

Senior American officials convinced themselves that the standard public health response to an outbreak of influenza should provide the basis of the response to coronavirus. On 27 February, health and human services secretary Alex Azar told the House Committee on Ways and Means that 'the immediate risk to the public remains low … [coronavirus] will look and feel to the American people more like a severe flu season in terms of the interventions and approaches you will see'. Azar said that it was 'unlikely that large numbers of Americans would need to be hospitalised as a result of coronavirus infection'.[9]

The American politicisation of the coronavirus response swiftly encompassed not only China but also the WHO. At a time when the WHO should have been focused entirely on supporting a unified global response to coronavirus, its gearing-up was greatly impeded by a campaign of political intimidation confected by the Trump administration. From February 2020 onwards, the world's ability to respond effectively to COVID-19 was crippled by the triumph of political imperatives over public health considerations.

The twin dead weights of politics and poor pandemic planning played out over February and March. The United States sank into anti-science denialism and institutional incompetence driven by the overwhelming political requirements and calculations of president Trump. The consequence of this was that the United States let coronavirus in.

In contrast, Hong Kong, Taiwan, Singapore and Vietnam led mostly Asian countries in closing borders, implementing quarantine and testing regimes, and mobilising their peoples and institutions to repel COVID-19. The responses of the rest of the world, including Australia, played out along the spectrum between 'pure politics' and 'pure public health'.

THE RIGHT PLAN FOR THE WRONG VIRUS

In Australia, as in the United States, national pandemic planning had been constructed around an influenza paradigm. It was the right plan for the wrong virus. The news from China should have caused every country, including Australia, that had based its pandemic planning on that paradigm to review and revise their plans. It was obvious that what was on the way was a SARS1-type virus.

Australia and New Zealand had two invaluable structural advantages on their side: geography and the internet. As remote Southern Hemisphere island nations, their geographical isolation conferred the benefit of time. The virus could only spread as fast as people could travel. Australia and New Zealand were not on the main global trade and tourist routes along which coronavirus began to spread from late 2019. Commendably, on 1 February 2020, Australia stopped direct air travel to/from China and subsequently Iran and South Korea. The virus would have to arrive indirectly through Europe, North America or other Asian ports. And while the virus travelled at the speed of an aircraft, information about the nature of coronavirus out of China, and elsewhere, travelled at the speed of light. The question for both Australia and New Zealand was whereabouts on the band between 'Let it in' and 'Keep it out' they would choose to land.

As the first reports came out of China in November and December 2019, I took more than a passing interest in what was going on. Through my involvement with HIV/AIDS, I had seen the chaos which had engulfed communities and governments around the world as they struggled to make sense of the sudden emergence of a new and deadly disease. I had witnessed the destructive political chicanery that had played out around the emergence of HIV/AIDS. Politicisation of the HIV response had transformed a serious but manageable problem into a global pandemic. When coronavirus emerged, I assumed that the work of those times would have been built on to strengthen Australia's response.

The Australian public health system had responded superbly to HIV/AIDS and to every viral threat and challenge since then. Surely, I thought, the lessons had been well learned. The public health principles and structures that had been developed and applied so well for so long would again be arrayed against this new viral challenge. Now, as in the days of HIV/AIDS, I expected public health to be prioritised over party politics. But at the back of my mind, I had my doubts.

As we swung into the new year, there were more pressing things to think about. Since July 2019, New South Wales had been affected by the worst bushfires in living memory. That December, Sydney was not the carefree, hedonistic city that it usually was in the lead-up to Christmas. The choking, acrid smoke did not lift as the weeks wore on but settled over the city like a funeral shroud. A few days after the subdued New Year's Eve celebrations, I left Sydney for London. It was a relief to arrive in a cold, sunny and wintry city, and for the first time in weeks to be able to breathe cool, clean air rather than suffering from the crippling effects of smoke inhalation.

During January 2020, I followed the emerging response of the UK Government to the news from China. There seemed to be little concern or urgency, even as the scope of the emergency widened dramatically. There was, for example, no interest in restricting or stopping travel from China into the United Kingdom. Media reports explained that the reason for this otherwise inexplicably passive approach was that the UK Government was basing its response on the principles of herd immunity. The combination of general herd immunity, development of annual vaccines and wide immunisation generally keeps rates of illness and deaths from influenza at very low levels, depending on the severity of annual strains. But from my experience of HIV/AIDS, I knew enough about viruses to know that there is a great difference between those that cause influenza, SARS1 and HIV.

The effect of adopting a herd immunity response can be summarised in the phrase 'Let it in and let it run'. Over time, the virus will infect the population at large. In theory, generally older people and those with weaker immune systems will fall ill and some will die. Thereby, according to Darwinian principles, the strong survive and, over time, the immunity of the 'herd' will be built up. Herd immunity requires exposure of an entire population to a virus. For long-established viruses such as influenza, we have vaccines that, over time, are administered and build up this herd immunity. New strains require new vaccines, but these are administered into a population with general immunity and therefore transmission rates, illnesses and deaths are kept low.

So by definition, there can be no herd immunity for a highly contagious new virus like coronavirus. As at October 2020, there is no vaccine. No country has had more than a very small fraction of its population exposed to the virus, and on the basis of less than a year's experience, nothing conclusive is known about the consequences of infection and the likelihood of reinfection by coronavirus. Yet in the United Kingdom, the chief medical and scientific advisers to the government, Chris Whitty and Patrick Vallance, were strenuously advocating herd immunity as the appropriate response to the emerging viral challenge.

On 20 April 2020, *The Times* of London published an investigative report into the early months of the UK Government's response to coronavirus. The report stated that 'all of the planning was for pandemic flu', and it made it clear that the UK's key advisers were, from the end of January, 'absolutely focused' on herd immunity They rejected the Asian view that the disease was along the lines of SARS, which required an immediate lockdown.[10]

From London, I also kept abreast of the Australian Government's response to the coronavirus emergency. By the first week of February, when I returned to Australia, it was obvious that coronavirus had spread into major cities in Asia. Recalling the days of SARS1,

I expected that, in transit through Singapore and on arrival in Sydney, I would find that the same sorts of measures that had been taken at the time of SARS1 had been implemented to deal with coronavirus. Indeed, on arrival at Singapore, passengers on my flight were temperature-checked both on disembarking the London flight and leaving for Sydney. I fully expected that when I arrived in Sydney on 4 February, I would also at least have to pass through temperature-checking and some form of screening.

Surprisingly, no such measures were in place at Sydney Airport. Was this just a matter of the bureaucracy taking a few days to catch up with the realities of a very fast-moving situation? Or was it a matter of policy?

On 7 February, the Australian Department of Health released the *Australian Health Sector Emergency Response Plan for Novel Coronavirus (COVID-19)*. I consulted the plan for guidance and reassurance about how the Australian Government and its advisers intended to approach the looming pandemic. At first glance, it appeared to be comprehensive and well considered. It identified the key strategic and organisational steps necessary to deal with the threat posed by coronavirus. But on my second reading, I began to wonder if it might not be a plan for the wrong virus. On the very first page of the *Emergency Response Plan*, the executive summary spoke of the threat of pandemic influenza. Nowhere was there a clear statement that coronavirus was in fact very different to the influenza virus and it might therefore require a very different set of responses. Even more disturbingly, the term 'proportionate' was used repeatedly to characterise the Australian pandemic response.

'Proportionate' meant letting the virus in and only then dealing with its effects. 'Proportionate' is not 'Prevention'.

During February, the world was transfixed by the unedifying spectacle of the *Diamond Princess*. The cruise ship had docked in Yokohama with some cases of coronavirus infection among its 3700 passengers and crew. However, the Japanese authorities obliged the passengers and crew to stay on the vessel for a two-week quarantine rather than be distributed around hospitals in Japan. Completely predictably, confining all those on board meant that the infection spread throughout the vessel. By the end of the botched quarantine, some 700 people had been infected. The vulnerability of cruise ships to coronavirus and the threat that it posed to passengers, crew and healthcare workers prompted the government of Taiwan to cease all cruise ship calls and activity in its waters from 6 February.

Apparently ignoring the wisdom of this decision, Australian authorities made no move to stop cruise ships calling at local ports. Many public health experts privately shared my concern and dismay. I was told their views had been expressed to responsible senior officers in the Commonwealth and state departments of health.

They had also been expressed to at least some of those who had been appointed to the so-called Australian Health Protection Principal Committee (AHPCC).

The AHPCC comprised the Commonwealth, state and territory chief medical officers and others. However, beyond these ex-officio appointments, the other members of the AHPCC were not disclosed. Other subcommittees had been constituted but their memberships were also secret. I have been around long enough in Australian politics to know one thing about secrecy. If the membership, proceedings and advice of committees are kept secret, it is because those who establish such bodies seek to avoid responsibility and accountability for their decisions and advice. The development of public health policy in Australia had never before been subordinate to the national security processes of the Australian Government. But now, the entire structure of the AHPCC's advice had been constituted under the National Security Committee of Cabinet. The minister for health was not a member of the National Security Committee.

A culture of secrecy is completely antithetical to the notion of public health policymaking and implementation. Success in creating good public health policies and measures rests entirely on a foundation of science, facts and evidence. If science is to be effective in informing public policy in time to contain or prevent the spread of a viral pandemic, the rapid, free and unimpeded flow of information, findings, facts and evidence is essential. Over that February, there should have been a full and open debate about the plans proposed by the Australian Government to deal with coronavirus.

In fact, the Australian medical advisers had settled on a small group of 'peer' countries with whom they were in regular contact, the most important of which were the United Kingdom and the United States. Collectively, the United Kingdom, the United States and Australia appeared to be working together and responding as if the threat was from influenza rather than something akin to SARS. This obviated the need to implement stringent border measures to stop the entry of COVID-19 into these countries. Rather, applying the influenza paradigm meant that they could take time to detect outbreaks and respond to them. There was a settled belief that there was no need for en-masse testing to detect asymptomatic carriers, no need to proceed to general lockdown arrangements, and no need to mandate the use of masks or implement stringent social distancing measures. And, evidently in the interests of not creating public concern or alarm, it was decided that there was no need for communication and education campaigns to advise the public about the looming threat and to begin the process of changing risky behaviours.

Adopting the influenza paradigm meant that the public health advice going to governments pressed for a slow, balanced approach. It also conformed with the interests of the governments of the United Kingdom and the United States, which were both under pressure to avoid action that would seriously affect economic activity. The difference was between 'let it in' and 'keep it out'. In the United Kingdom, the United States and Australia, the watchword was 'proportionate'—managing but not preventing the spread of coronavirus was the policy.

SECRET HEALTH

On 25 January 2020, the first Australian case of coronavirus infection was recorded, in Melbourne. However, in the subsequent three weeks or so, almost no other Australians contracted COVID-19, apart from those unfortunate enough to have been trapped on board the *Diamond Princess*. The lack of local cases detracted from any sense of urgency in contemplating what should be done after the imposition of the direct travel ban from China on 1 February.

The proportionate approach dovetailed neatly with the political imperatives of the Commonwealth, state and territory governments. So at the top political levels, there was no appetite or inclination on the part of leaders to challenge the assumptions and consequences of this strategy. After the recent disastrous bushfires, governments were preoccupied with rebuilding the tourist trade in Australia, not with taking measures to diminish it. Indeed, in February, the governments of Queensland and the Northern Territory both launched international tourist campaigns—this at a time when the virus spread to at least seventy-five countries, with thousands of cases reported in nations as different as Iran, South Korea and Italy.

Australia has many excellent public health professionals, especially at the state/territory level, where responsibility lies for local hospitals, clinics and other health facilities. They were well aware of the pressing need to take action to deal with the coming wave of coronavirus infections. Across the nation, including throughout the health system, there was rising concern, discussion and much precautionary activity, at least at the operational level. And so, at the beginning of February, it seemed to me improbable that Australian public health authorities genuinely subscribed to the notion of herd immunity. But the concept was mentioned publicly by several members of the AHPCC. In interviews, they said they expected that somewhere between 20 per cent and 70 per cent of the population would be infected by coronavirus. Their concern was to ensure that the growth of cases was staggered so as to prevent hospital intensive care beds from being overwhelmed.

Perhaps I had misunderstood what was going on or what was being said. I thought it best to go to the source of these figures, which had been reported as the modelling conducted by the Doherty Institute in Melbourne. From my days dealing with HIV/AIDS, I knew that such modelling should not be taken to be a prediction as to how an epidemic would progress. But no matter how long and hard (naive) modellers remind their customers that their endeavours are not predictive, politicians are irresistibly tempted to latch onto whichever of the three standard scenarios (bad, the same, better) best suit their political purposes. For politicians, modelling is prediction by another name. Whatever the scenarios that were being outlined for coronavirus, I knew how critical it was for the assumptions that underpinned the scenario planning to be clearly spelled out, interrogated and justified.

If the government was being told that an infection rate of at least 20 per cent of the population was inevitable, then it was a matter of the utmost gravity, not to mention democratic principle, that the assumptions about what type of virus was being planned for, and what alternatives existed, should be up for searching analysis and review. However, all the papers commissioned from Australian research institutes and all the deliberations and advice being provided by the AHPCC were secret and unavailable for public debate and discussion. In the critical early days of formulating the Australian response to the most serious and dangerous public health threat in a century, the planning and preparations were a state secret, and the lines of authority, responsibility and accountability of those advising Australian governments were unknown and confidential.

Public health had never been and cannot be secret health. It was hard to square the tone of complacency and managerial invincibility with the accelerating global spread of the virus.

The official words of calm reassurance were clearly not mollifying the Australian people. The most obvious sign of increasing public concern was the widespread panic buying of essentials, notably toilet paper, that swept Australia in late February.[11] There is no doubt as to why this panic buying erupted. On Monday 24 February, after holding up for almost two weeks longer than Wall Street, the Australian stock market began one of the most severe declines in its history. The collapse was a critical turning point in the public's concern about the threat posed by coronavirus. Australians were rapidly developing a more urgent understanding of the gravity of the situation than their government and its advisers.

The light and slow approach of the Australian Government made no sense to a public justifiably alarmed by reports of the spread of the virus into Europe and the breakdown of financial markets. This cognitive dissonance was also apparent in the United Kingdom and the United States. Whether for reasons of international diplomacy or because they genuinely did not consider their countries to be at risk, during February the US, UK and Australian governments had consulted with each other and shipped to China very large quantities of personal protective equipment (PPE) from their national stockpiles.

By any rational calculation, the month of February should have been devoted to urgent strengthening of Australia's defences against the impending threat. Stocks of PPE should have been increased rather than run down. Border surveillance should have been implemented. Travel restrictions should have been placed on travel not just from China, Iran and South Korea but from Europe generally and North America. The operations of cruise ships should have been suspended. Parliament and the people should have been methodically informed about the deteriorating situation globally and what Australian authorities were planning.

The basic assumptions that underpinned the national pandemic plan should have been opened to debate and subjected to contestability and criticism. The entire pandemic plan should have been recast in light of the rapidly changing evidence and facts.

NOT BUSINESS AS USUAL

My apprehension about the perplexing failure of the Australian authorities to prepare for the pandemic came to a head when the Sydney Gay and Lesbian Mardi Gras took place. On the evening of Saturday 29 February, I joined the many tens of thousands of participants, spectators, revellers and partygoers thronging the streets and clubs of the inner city. Touring the highways and byways of Sydney on the Mardi Gras weekend confirmed just how many tourists were in town. But I could not reconcile how it could be possible to bring together hundreds of thousands of people in Sydney while a global pandemic involving a new and dangerous infectious disease was daily gathering strength and speed.

At the end of that weekend, I was convinced that it would have been far better had the festival not taken place. Mardi Gras crystallised the doubts that had been growing in my mind since I had returned from London through the open-to-the-virus border at Sydney Airport. Certainly, if I had known then what was coming just weeks later, I would not have attended the festival. The Mardi Gras weekend demonstrated how easy it was to go on with business as usual, to ignore the speed at which events were moving. There was too much talking and not enough action. I was faced with the famous Groucho Marx question: 'Who are you going to believe? Me, or the evidence of your lying eyes?'

I decided to believe my eyes and to speak up. On 6 March 2020, *The Sydney Morning Herald* published my op-ed 'Our HIV Lesson: Exclude Politicians and Trust the Experts—and the People—to Confront Coronavirus'. That precipitated intense media interest and in subsequent months I appeared on many television programs, including *Q+A*, *Four Corners*,

60 Minutes, *7.30* and *The Project*, and major radio networks. My Twitter followers grew from eleven to over 21 000. The core of my argument was that public mobilisation around prevention was far preferable to waiting to see what happened, and only then to act. Slow and proportionate measures after the virus had arrived could never be as effective as stopping the virus at the borders. It was better not to let it in, but if it did enter, we had to take every necessary step to smash it.

After Mardi Gras, the next large-scale gathering attracting both domestic and international visitors was the Australian Formula One Grand Prix, scheduled to be held over the weekend of 14–15 March in Melbourne. It was obvious that to hold the grand prix would invite the risk of coronavirus transmission among the thousands of attendees. The battle lines were drawn between the commercial and media interests who insisted that the event proceed, and a wide range of independent experts who wanted it cancelled. The federal government and its advisers took the side of the organisers, wishing for it to go ahead, even though this made no public health sense. On his arrival in Melbourne, even the star racing driver Lewis Hamilton expressed his astonishment and concern that the grand prix was on, not off. Finally, on the morning of Friday 13 March, after ticket-holders had been waiting two hours for the gates to the race-track to open, Victorian Premier Daniel Andrews did the right thing and cancelled the event.

The evident confusion between Victorian and Commonwealth health advisers and political leaders only underscored the general lack of consultation and coordination between governments. The Australian federal system had become another impediment to dealing with coronavirus before it became a major public health problem.

The index of success in public health is the number of illnesses and deaths averted by preventive actions— or, if disease has taken hold, the pace at which rates of infection and death are reduced and the disease eliminated. For many politicians, however, success is measured in ratings, clicks, and how they come across on the evening news bulletins. Politics is the art of splitting the difference, compromise and putting off decisions likely to be unpopular. But the tension between the imperatives of public health and party politics cannot be resolved by splitting the difference. When a potentially catastrophic new viral threat emerges, the protection of public health requires that disruptive decisions, grounded in science and evidence, be taken immediately. And, of course, politicians in the end have to be accountable for decisions and their outcomes.

Behind the scenes, politicians' responsibilities are to convene, interrogate all advice, set strategic goals, and fund whatever is necessary in order to reduce and eliminate harm and disruption. It was worrying to see that, in the Australian response, politics had prevailed over public health.

On 2 March, Australia recorded its first case of community transmission, as distinct from cases involving travellers returning from overseas. From that time, the official Australian strategy was increasingly hampered by the strategy laid out in the *Emergency Response Plan*. Its assumptions about a proportionate response could not realistically apply to the facts of the spread of the virus during early March. Furthermore, the infection-control provisions made no reference to the possibility or desirability for the entire population to go into lockdown (as happened less than four weeks after the *Emergency Response Plan* was finally activated by the Prime Minister on 27 February). The term 'lockdown' was not in official favour within the AHPCC or the National Security Committee.

And while the infection-control guidelines referred to the need for respiratory hygiene and handwashing, there was no mention of the use of masks to reduce infection risk. Indeed, the dominant faction of infectious diseases advisers on the AHPCC was adamant in claiming that the use of masks in situations of elevated risk of transmission would do more harm than good. These advisers held to a longstanding academic view that respiratory infections were much more likely to be spread by physical contact than through tiny airborne droplets. As the weeks went on, however, it became clear that this advice also reflected the politics around the lack of stockpiling of adequate numbers of masks, and the decision to deplete the stockpile as late as February.

The need for 'border measures' to be reassessed was identified, but the potential total closing of borders was not. The *Emergency Response Plan* did not envisage that any overarching response would be required that involved the entire Australian population taking unprecedented measures to contain a pandemic threat. Yet Australia was moving inexorably towards the imposition of disruption on an immense scale. The tone of the *Emergency Response Plan* was to think and act small, not big.

An accelerating tempo of preparation and activity began taking place at the state and territory levels, as well as in the federal government. But over the first two weeks of March, what should have been a coordinated, countrywide response driven by the national government began to fragment between the states and territories. At the top level, the Australian Government was communicating using the tools of a bygone age— daily media conferences reported by the Canberra press gallery, carried on television networks and published in the next day's newspapers. Meanwhile, most of the Australian people, and especially young people, were sourcing news and views about coronavirus in real time through Facebook, Google News, Apple News, TikTok, Snapchat, Instagram and Twitter, and from relatively few mainstream online sites, of which the most authoritative and widely respected by far were those produced by the Australian Broadcasting Corporation. The old model of top-down, ex-cathedra communications had been made redundant by the rise of social media and a more connected population. Every day brought forth further confusion and increasingly contradictory statements from national, state and territorial leaders and their medical and scientific advisers.

The first contract for a national public information campaign was only put out to tender on 6 March. Work was commenced on a COVID contact-tracing app, which was released on 26 April, but it proved to be not as effective as manual tracing. More worrying was how the *Emergency Response Plan* had described an alphabet soup of subcommittees and tried to encompass every relevant department and agency, while creating an ad-hoc body—the AHPCC—with zero transparency and an apparent monopoly on advice given to the National Security Committee of Cabinet, but bypassing the health minister and their department.

The consequences of the poor structuring of the response played out in what can now be seen as the critical three weeks leading up to the national lockdown on 22 March. The advisers had failed to account for the speed at which the virus was spreading and the panic this would provoke. The commitment to 'proportionate' and a measured response was at odds with the inchoate but real expectation of the Australian people that the virus be stopped at the borders.

THE IDE(A)S OF MARCH

The exponential spread of the pandemic in Europe from mid-February provoked a searching reassessment by the United Kingdom of the coronavirus planning undertaken by its chief advisers, Chris Whitty and Patrick Vallance. Subsequent criticisms of the planning brought into full view the essential elements of the arguments that have since bedevilled the public debate about the response.

According to a Reuters special report, the UK Government's Scientific Advisory Group for Emergencies (SAGE) dug in against implementing a national lockdown: 'On March 12 came a bombshell for the British public. Chris Whitty, the chief medical officer, announced Britain had moved the threat to UK citizens from "moderate" to "high"'. Whitty confirmed that slowing the spread of coronavirus, rather than extinguishing it, was now the priority: 'It is no longer necessary for us to identify every case.'[12] Meanwhile, Vallance, who chaired SAGE, said in a radio interview on 13 March that the plan was to simply control the pace of infection. The government had, for now, rejected what Vallance called 'eye-catching measures' like stopping mass gatherings such as football games or closing schools. The 'aim is to try and reduce the peak, broaden the peak, not to suppress it completely'. Most people would get the virus mildly, and this would build up 'herd immunity' which, in time, would 'stop the disease's progress'.[13]

The advisers had deluded themselves that this approach could be adopted without public or parliamentary debate, sold to their political masters and implemented methodically and calmly. They were mistaken. It was the high point of the herd immunity construction, which almost immediately collapsed.

On 16 March, Professor Neil Ferguson and his colleagues at Imperial College London published a report that graphically forecast the consequences in the United Kingdom, ranging from uncontrolled spread (510 000 deaths) to what was termed 'mitigation' (250 000 deaths).[14] It was not that the Imperial College London paper did not reflect the secret modelling commissioned by the committees. The difference was that the paper put these alarming figures out into the public domain, unchecked and unfiltered by the official lines of advice and orthodoxy. It forced the UK Government to abandon its insouciant, laissez-faire policymaking. In Australia, the Imperial College London paper would have much the same impact.

After the decision to stop the grand prix, Prime Minister Morrison and his senior advisers dug in behind their policy prescriptions, even though public opinion was rapidly shifting away from an automatic acceptance that the government was ahead of developments and in control of the situation. On Friday

13 March, the Prime Minister attempted to minimise the news of the grand prix cancellation by declaring that he would, the next day, be attending a National Rugby League match in suburban Sydney. This came after several instances in the previous week where the Prime Minister and his chief advisers had made public displays of handshaking and downplaying the need for social distancing. At his press conference, in line with the proportionate strategies of the *Emergency Response Plan*, Prime Minister Morrison also foreshadowed that in the coming week, consideration would be given to limiting gatherings of over 500 people, and some other related measures.

People listen to prime ministers. On the cusp of a pandemic that would be caused in Australia by infections that were already present but undetected in Sydney and Melbourne, it seemed to me the height of irresponsibility for the Prime Minister to attend a gathering of thousands of people, ignoring the need for social distancing. This behaviour would send a message to the public that things were not as bad as was being made out.

Later that evening, Prime Minister Morrison backtracked on his intention to attend the match. Why was it right to commit to attending the game in the afternoon but decide not to attend it only hours later? The events of that fateful Friday confirmed that the Commonwealth Government and its advisers were committed to policies, derived from the United

Kingdom, that if implemented would inevitably have serious repercussions for Australian public health.

The implosion of the main bulwarks of the *Emergency Response Plan* in the week of 15 March had at least three major causes:

- the release on 16 March of the Imperial College London paper that blew the whistle on the modelling that had hitherto been kept secret in the United Kingdom and Australia
- rising levels of public concern about coronavirus infection evidenced by panic buying; the accelerating collapse of financial markets; and saturation reporting of the exponential growth of coronavirus cases, especially in Italy and South Korea
- the increasingly confusing series of announcements by federal authorities on banning gatherings of various sizes, social distancing measures, the closing of ever-changing lists of businesses, and a steadfast refusal to countenance nationwide lockdowns and school closures.

The virus was now well established in Australia. Over the second week of March, Australia's reported case load began to increase exponentially, reflecting the rise in case numbers in Italy in the preceding weeks.

In contrast to the uncertainty that had engulfed the federal government's public statements, the Australian business community had begun to move definitively against the threat. From mid-February, many large

Australian businesses and institutions began to allow their staff to work from home. This advice did not apply to all workers in all situations, but it effectively began to reduce density and possible transmission by emptying out the large office towers in the central business districts of cities and towns, and greatly reducing public transport use to and from those areas. These unprecedented measures were dictated not just by the nature of the public health emergency but also by increased public apprehension, which was already at a very high level. The federal government was falling well behind the rising public and business concern, which was being registered by state and territory governments and leaders.

In a series of press conferences, Prime Minister Morrison and his advisers struggled to explain the rationale for step-by-step, proportionate measures around restrictions on gatherings and recommended business closures. Behind the scenes—and sometimes in front of them—Australian governments began to disagree and diverge over the most effective response to the peril. Public opinion had moved decisively in favour of an immediate lockdown. But the Australian Government was stubbornly unwilling to move until more cases of the virus had emerged. It was still adhering to the inevitability, if not the desirability, of 'letting it in and letting it run'.

On 12 March, it was publicly confirmed by the AHPCC that the Doherty Institute's confidential modelling stated that '20 percent, or around 1.5 million NSW residents, would be infected in the "first wave" of the virus'.[15] The publication of the Imperial College London paper dealt the final blow to the Australian Government's attempt to corral state and territory governments within the slow and proportionate strategy. This added further fuel to the long-overdue public debate that had broken out between politicians, experts, commentators and critics. The assumptions and consequences of the pandemic planning under-taken behind closed doors were, more or less, exposed to public view, criticism and debate in mid-March, after the virus had already entered the country. It became apparent to the leaders of the states and territories, though not to the national leadership, that Australia must move into full lockdown.

On 20 March, Tasmania announced that it would close its borders. Then the premiers of New South Wales and Victoria blindsided the Prime Minister and announced that their states would immediately move into lockdown. The remaining states and terri-tories followed suit. By 22 March, all hope of a single national response aimed at preventing the spread of coronavirus was lost.

While it was not apparent at the time, the states and territories had to one degree or another opted to take the stringent measures required to eliminate further transmission of the virus, to test and trace all cases of the virus that had entered their jurisdictions, and to maintain the lockdowns for three cycles of the virus. They did so against the advice and wishes of the national government but with the full support of their citizens.

The aim of the strategy should have been 'Don't let it in', taking all measures necessary to bring about zero local transmission of the virus. The various governments elected by the people of Australia, and those of New Zealand, had now embarked on a real-time experiment to determine which measures might best contain and possibly eliminate local transmission.

THE FRACTURED RESPONSE

By 1 February 2020, all the necessary scientific information about coronavirus was well known to international agencies, national governments and expert institutions, and was largely in the public domain. Armed with this knowledge, some countries moved swiftly to recast their previous pandemic plans and take all the steps necessary to halt the spread of coronavirus across their borders. These countries correctly understood that they were dealing with a variant of SARS, not a variant of influenza. As soon as their responses were activated, comprehensive public communications and education were undertaken.

Vietnam, with its long land border with China, and also Taiwan are outstanding models of effective and comprehensive public health responses to coronavirus.

Vietnam, a lower-income country but with a robust
socialist public health system, instituted lockdowns.
Taiwan never closed its schools and businesses but
ramped up its testing and contact-tracing regimes,
increased mask production, and offered generous
financial support to all workers exposed to or afflicted
by coronavirus.

Other countries, including the United Kingdom
and Australia, did not recast their plans, nor did they
deviate from the basic principles and assumptions
underlying their pandemic planning. Australian
authorities did not seem greatly concerned with the
precautionary measures being taken to the north.
Vietnam, Taiwan, Thailand and other Asian countries
were not regarded as peer countries and therefore
were presumably not consulted in the critical weeks
of January and February 2020, nor have they been
since. It also is not known whether, during that
time, Australian authorities were in continuing and
meaningful direct contact with Chinese medical
and scientific agencies and authorities. The United
Kingdom, in contrast, was held by the AHPCC to be a
peer country despite embarking on a catastrophically
ill-conceived path to disaster.

By mid-March, the crisis could no longer be
ignored, despite the evident reluctance to take
precipitate actions that might impinge on business
activity or confidence. Under immense pressure, the
Australian Government abandoned the key elements

of the strategy developed by its advisers from January 2020, and based on the concept of herd immunity as derived from the influenza paradigm. By that time, the consequences of confusion and poor planning were becoming obvious.

THE *RUBY PRINCESS*

On 19 March, the cruise ship *Ruby Princess* docked in Sydney, and passengers exposed to or infected with coronavirus were allowed to disembark before testing results had been received—events that exposed the weaknesses of Australia's pandemic planning. What went wrong was forensically laid out in the report of the Special Commission of Inquiry into the Ruby Princess brought down by special commissioner Bret Walker SC on 14 August 2020.[16] At least twenty-eight deaths and 662 coronavirus cases were linked to the cruise ship. In his report, Walker found that there had been serious, inexcusable and inexplicable mistakes made in the handling of the vessel's arrival in Sydney. But even so, the commissioner broadly found that the individuals involved had acted within their remits and to the best of their knowledge and abilities. The *Ruby Princess* disaster was not so much the fault of the individuals tasked with carrying out this or that function. Rather, the disaster had its genesis in the complex, contradictory and fundamentally unworkable nature of the *Emergency Response Plan*.

The *Emergency Response Plan* struck a compromise between the two levels of government and between the many agencies and departments involved in one way or another with what might be thought to be the relatively straightforward business of managing cruise ship arrivals and departures. In normal times, these arrangements worked smoothly. But by mid-March, normal times had passed. The saga of the *Ruby Princess*'s sister ship, the *Diamond Princess*, had already highlighted the very serious threat posed to cruise ships by coronavirus. By mid-February at the latest, Australia should have followed Taiwan's example earlier that month and stopped all cruise ship activity at Australian ports. Yet no such decision was taken.

The secrecy under which the deliberations of the AHPCC is cloaked means that we have no idea if the committee considered halting cruise ship operations; what, if any, recommendation it made to federal ministers; and whether ministers accepted or rejected any advice given by the AHPCC. The Australian Government refused to provide documents or to allow its officers to appear at the special commission. The *Diamond Princess* event does not appear to have triggered any overhaul or review of the mechanisms by which cruise ship arrivals were to be handled under the arrangements laid down in the national plan.

The *Emergency Response Plan* created a web of arrangements that so distributed responsibility and accountability that no one agency or individual could take the decisions necessary to protect the health and wellbeing of the passengers and crew on the *Ruby Princess*, much less public health, once they had disembarked.

THE END OF CONSENSUS

The aim of creating one national strategic response to coronavirus broke down on 22 March when the premiers of New South Wales and Victoria forced the national lockdown on an unwilling and reluctant federal government. It came at just about the last possible moment to avoid far more serious consequences. Only a lockdown could break the chain of transmission. The Australian public saw what was happening in Italy and the United States and grasped this simple proposition. They wished to keep the virus out. Yet, at the top political level, this step had been resisted.

While it was little appreciated at the time, the fracturing of the national response created, on the Australian continent and New Zealand, seven separate real-time experiments: in New South Wales/Victoria/the Australian Capital Territory, then Queensland, Western Australia, Tasmania, South Australia, the Northern Territory and New Zealand. In seven Petri dishes, covering a combined population of some thirty million people, significantly different assumptions and goals regarding how best to manage coronavirus were being put into practice.

At one end of the spectrum, New Zealand chose the goal of ending local community transmission by imposing very stringent lockdown provisions. These were significantly harsher than those adopted by Australian governments. The key New Zealand decision had been to set a time-limited target for the elimination of local transmission and then to mobilise all necessary resources to achieve the target. New Zealand's advisers, led by Professor Michael Baker, assumed, as had their counterparts in Taiwan and Vietnam, that this was a realistic and achievable goal given what was known about the nature of the coronavirus.

At the other end of the spectrum was the Australian Government, whose advisers privately and publicly rejected the New Zealand model.

At the end of March, the AHPCC grudgingly accepted the inevitability of the lockdown that they had opposed, and the term 'herd immunity' was successively rebadged variously as 'mitigation', 'living with the virus', 'COVID normal' and 'aggressive suppression'. The group of advisers in and around the AHPCC who had devised the original strategy buttressed their efforts to persuade their political masters and the mainstream press of their correctness. However, the strategic writ of the AHPCC had ceased to apply in much of the country.

Once they shut their borders, Australia's states and territories began to organise around the goal of eliminating local community transmission. Over April and May, almost all moved to increase their investments in testing and contact tracing, greatly strengthened the quarantine reception arrangements for returning citizens, and increased the supply of PPE for use in hospitals and clinics.

The Australian people had come to the settled view that the best way to live with COVID-19 was to live without it. These efforts paid off in dramatic falls in new cases over the period of the March–May lockdown.

DOWN TO ZERO

The most adroit and successful effort to square political and public health imperatives came in New South Wales, which had entered the 2020 pandemic with considerable advantages insofar as its public health structures were concerned. From the 1980s, New South Wales had rebuilt and expanded its public health structures to handle the complex prevention, care and treatment demands of the HIV/AIDS pandemic. Successive governments greatly increased the state's public health budgets and expertise at all levels. New South Wales also developed and implemented a decentralised structure for running its health system based on fifteen Local Health Districts (LHDs), with well-resourced local Public Health Units capable of supporting local staff and patient case loads. These LHDs were centred on local hospitals, but not to the point of ceding to these hospitals control over the vital functions of public health outreach and management.

For some four decades, ministers and heads of NSW Health had progressively reinforced the role of public health within the overall health system. The legislation governing public health in New South Wales was developed and refined to establish clear lines of responsibility and accountability for the chief health officer, who was appointed at the appropriately senior deputy secretary level, reporting directly to the secretary and the minister for health. The need to involve and connect with communities to promote and pursue public health objectives was another core principle. Fortified by the robustness of this structure, New South Wales in effect pursued the goal of eliminating local transmission, and to their credit, local authorities had the resolve and humility to learn the right lessons from the *Ruby Princess* episode. Testing and contact-tracing measures were rapidly improved and brought to scale. The administration of quarantine and self-isolation arrangements was upgraded. The results were striking. By the end of May, New South Wales had brought recorded local transmissions down to zero, and it maintained this level for some three weeks.

Similar success was obtained in all the other states and territories. Those Australian and New Zealand jurisdictions that began 2020 with robust, well-funded public health systems, built around the principles of collective action and community involvement, were far better placed to deal with the arrival of coronavirus than those jurisdictions that did not. They adopted wholeheartedly the goal of eliminating local transmissions, and overall, the success of the national lockdown rapidly became obvious. By the end of April, new cases plateaued at about seventy reported cases a day, and then began to decline to an average of about twenty new cases a day by the beginning of May. Supported by the availability of more and better test kits, the eligibility criteria for testing were widened in an effort to locate and deal with hidden cases of community transmission.

The success of the March–May lockdown was down to the common sense and good judgement of the Australian people, channelled for the most part properly and well through the political leaders who were closest to them—the premiers and chief ministers. The lockdown was then put into effect by the hundreds of thousands of citizens who comprise the Australian healthcare sector and the essential workforce.

The pandemic and associated economic troubles had crashed over an Australia that was unprepared for the double dumper. But the lockdown worked. By early June, Australia had secured impressive outcomes that mirrored those of New Zealand while not having imposed as stringent a lockdown. In less than three months, by applying and sustaining the simplest of behavioural changes, the Australian people had dissipated the immediate danger of a coronavirus pandemic. The great self-organising collective that is the

Australian public health system had asserted itself over the directions and expectations of the high command.

The Australian states and territories and New Zealand had, both by design and accident, uncovered how to sustainably all-but-eliminate local transmission of coronavirus. This involved closing borders to all non-essential travel and imposing a strict and effective set of quarantine and isolation arrangements on incoming travellers. Within those secured borders, a combination of social distancing, personal hygiene measures and disinfection of surfaces, and a three-cycle lockdown removed the virus from local circulation.

The achievements of the lockdown also demonstrated that, whatever the public health measures, they all had to be buttressed by money. Money is the greatest vaccine of all. It has always been the case that health outcomes are worse in the low-income and marginal groups in society. The richer and better off you are, the healthier you are likely to be. It is just the same, but only more so, in pandemics. Postcodes correlate very well with health outcomes. The poor and the marginal are faced with a real and cruel choice between protecting their health and ensuring their economic survival. Without governments aligning financial support for the most vulnerable with public health objectives, poor people have no choice but to place the short-term need to buy food and pay rent over their own and the community's interest in staving off infection.

The sense of relief at seeing off the threat of coronavirus obscured the fact that the modelling and assumptions relied upon by the AHPCC had not come to pass. The committee had been adamant that the Australian people would not accept a large-scale lockdown. Indeed, from the inception of the *Emergency Response Plan*, it appears that the AHPCC had been convinced that no lockdown could, would or should be used to stem the spread of coronavirus, and that therefore at best, coronavirus would infect some 20 per cent of the Australian population. No doubt to the astonishment of the AHPCC and the federal government, the one preventive measure that had never featured in their planning—the lockdown—was the one thing that worked splendidly to avert the catastrophe that, by 22 March, they expected was inevitable and unavoidable. Very stringent social movement restrictions were the only prudent and precautionary steps that should have been considered and recommended.

The scale of the health and economic packages announced in mid-March 2020 demonstrated that the government had expected the worst. In these packages, there were substantial provisions, such as the increase in JobSeeker payments and the introduction of JobKeeper wage subsidies, that bolstered the public health measures. But by excluding so-called gig-economy workers and obliging them to raid their retirement savings to survive, the government exacerbated a public health problem that would soon become apparent in Victoria. There were better alternatives than to throw millions into unemployment. The government went from complacency and proportionate response to the harshest and most sweeping measures, without ever stopping at the station marked 'lockdown'.

This failure had disastrous consequences. The massive economic dislocation and misery caused by mass unemployment, and the destruction of entire sectors of the economy, were predicated, in Australia at least, on wrong assumptions. The proper public health advice should have been that the arrival of coronavirus was serious but entirely manageable. There was not the slightest reason to do more in economic terms than to implement the short-term income and job-support measures that bolstered the behavioural changes required to see the virus off the premises. In most of Europe, apart from the chaotic shambles in the United Kingdom, the first wave of the pandemic was far more severe than it proved to be in Australia. Yet in no European country did the public health emergency also panic governments into such drastic and damaging economic and social upheavals as in Australia.

By the end of June, however, what had happened and why seemed to be of academic interest only. Buoyed by their apparent victory over the virus, the governments of Australia, their advisers and the public assumed that the worst was disappearing in the rear-view mirror. Under pressure from business, the federal

UNMASKED: THE POLITICS OF PANDEMICS

government asserted that it was time to open up, to hustle the Australian people out from under the doona and to get used to the new economic and social realities engineered by the sweeping reforms of a month earlier.

FREEDOM TO INFECT

The success of the lockdown unfortunately masked some serious structural deficiencies in the Victorian public health system, some of which were longstanding.

The Victorian public health system was organised around individual hospitals and not, as in New South Wales, around more diverse, community-based LHDs. At the outbreak of the pandemic, therefore, Victoria had strong central control and direction of policy. But in public health, as in life, you get what you pay for. In 2017–18, Australian health expenditure was $185 billion, including health spending by governments, individuals, insurers and other private sources. In that period, all Australian state and territory governments spent approximately 1 per cent of that figure—$1.39 billion—on public health, with the Victorian Government accounting for just $400 million of that, sums that are scarcely noticeable within the totality of Australian health budgets.[17] The chronic underfunding of public health meant that Victoria entered the pandemic lacking a large, well-organised and trained public health workforce able to rapidly assume responsibility for implementing the scaling up of contact tracing, testing, and quarantine surveillance and monitoring.

New South Wales had built on the public health structures established in response to HIV/AIDS. Victoria had let them atrophy. And it is extremely difficult to rebuild such structures when an emergency has already begun. The apparently successful outcomes achieved by June 2020 engendered complacency, obviating the need to look more closely and urgently at workforce and skill set gaps to avoid the second wave.

The inability of the Victorian Government to deal with resurgent infections was compounded by the emergence of a deeply irresponsible partisan political campaign launched under the rubric 'Freedom Day'. The campaign asserted that the lockdown had been a gross overreaction to the actual threat posed by coronavirus and an infringement of individuals' liberty. It provided an umbrella for several lines of attack on the lockdown strategy. First, academics and scientists aligned with the AHPCC strategy continued to claim that, as in Sweden, the spread of the virus should be accepted as a way to achieve herd immunity rather than rely on lockdowns. There was also relentless pressure from business interests, especially those involved in retailing, tourism and travel, to reignite demand for their products and services through the rapid reopening of their sectors. Finally, libertarian and fringe groups, inspired by their American counterparts, used the lockdown to question the stringency of the measures, the facts around COVID-19, and the value of science and expertise.

These various arguments were pursued by senior members of the Victorian Liberal Opposition and echoed, amplified and rehashed by elements in the mainstream media, including enthusiastic commentators for News Corp outlets. It was asserted that the lockdown was a plot to deprive people of their inalienable rights, one driven by the urge to create fear and panic rather than rely on 'facts' known only to those pushing these myths—not to science. These 'facts' would show that coronavirus was not nearly as problematic as had been claimed. There was, therefore, every reason to throw off the shackles, abandon the nonsense of behavioural measures to stem the risks of transmission, and return to 'normal'. The federal colleagues of the Victorian Liberal Opposition said nothing to rein in the puerility of these political attacks, and the line between public health and party politics began to blur.

As is often the case in electoral politics, the Freedom Day campaign was boosted by luck and chance. In Victoria, the onset of coronavirus exposed pre-existing weaknesses in public health structures and the management of contact tracing, quarantine and infection control in hospitals and aged-care facilities. The question of whether to support the lockdown had become not a matter of science but of party politics. The prudent public health measures adopted by the

Andrews government still enjoyed great public support, but somewhat less with each passing day. The evident success of the first lockdown in reducing daily case numbers to low double digits had contributed to the public's erroneous assumptions that the virus had been defeated.

This is the paradox of prevention. The lockdown in fact prevented matters from becoming far worse than they would have been had it never taken place or been imposed later than 22 March. One only had to look at the United States and the United Kingdom to see what might have happened in Australia had preventive action not been taken in time. Yet the proponents of Freedom Day cynically argued that the relatively low numbers of coronavirus cases at the end of the lockdown proved that the threat had never been that great in the first place.

The Victorian lockdown arrangements, along with those in New South Wales and other states, began to ease from mid-May, which in retrospect was too soon. Victoria had a consistent drumbeat of community transmissions that reflected shortcomings in the contact-tracing arrangements. But Freedom Day had been proclaimed. Its irresponsibility gave the Victorian people permission to wave farewell to the very real threat still posed by uncontained community transmission. On its front pages and in its editorials and opinion columns, *The Herald Sun* welcomed freedom from the 'tyranny' of Premier Andrews, who was caricatured as 'Dictator Dan'. And so, free to resume replication, the virus reasserted itself. As a creature of the laws of physics, chemistry and biology, the virus exploited the collapse of precautionary measures. Nemesis followed hubris.

The first sign that things were not going as they should in Victoria had come as early as 2 May with an outbreak at Cedar Meats in the Melbourne western suburb of Brooklyn. There had also been serious lapses in the security arrangements at several of Melbourne's quarantine hotels, the circumstances of which would become the subject of a board of inquiry two months later.[18] The Victorian case load rose rapidly, from only two cases on 7 June to seventy-six daily cases by the end of the month.

On 20 June, the Victorian Government embarked on the progressive tightening of restrictions on households, gatherings, and the operations of business. Local lockdowns were then expanded across twelve different Melbourne postcodes. The accelerating spread of the virus forced the state government to reimpose restrictions based on the 'hotspot' model still favoured by the advisers to the AHPCC, under which local outbreaks could be identified and controlled without the entire city reverting to lockdown. To work, it required high levels of very efficient testing and tracing, the rapid return of results, and scrupulous adherence to quarantine, isolation and movement restrictions. Without these conditions being met, the hotspot strategy could not succeed. It has been a catastrophic failure in the United Kingdom. Indeed, these sequential lockdowns and closures did nothing to get ahead of the pace at which the virus was spreading through Melbourne. It was the application in practice of the 'living with COVID-19' strategy that, from the earliest days of the crisis, had formed the basis of the AHPCC *Emergency Response Plan*. Public confidence fell as the daily total of new cases increased.

Victoria shifted from lockdown to Freedom Day without ever passing through an intermediate stage that should have, at the very least, involved the widespread use of masks to impede the transmission of coronavirus. The refusal of the AHPCC to recommend mask usage is one of the most absurd and concerning features of the entire official public health response in Australia. In Victoria, the relevant committee refused to advise the mandatory use of masks until it was overruled by Premier Andrews on 19 July.

The maintenance of free movement between Australia's two largest states had been a primary political objective of the federal government, central to its ambitions to proceed with an economic reopening before the virus had been eliminated. But, on 6 July, the New South Wales and Victorian governments announced that their shared border would shut. Victoria now had to deal with the second wave that had occurred because neither the federal government nor its own had absorbed the critical lessons of the first lockdown and the outcomes achieved in Australia's other states and territories, and in New Zealand. As in those jurisdictions, Victoria should have used the time afforded by the first lockdown to drastically overhaul and improve structures, personnel and procedures in regard to the core functions for which it had responsibility, and especially in relation to the prevention of infection in hospital settings.

THE AGED-CARE DEBACLE

In the provisions of the *Emergency Response Plan*, the protection of residents in aged-care facilities, and of health and aged-care workers, is accorded the highest priority. This is mentioned throughout the document, and the AHPCC, while it did not plan or intend a national lockdown, certainly understood that this was the core objective of the plan. It was entirely reasonable to expect that the federal government would apply all of its financial and organisational resources to buttress aged-care facilities against the spread of coronavirus, and to ensure that private operators took additional precautionary measures.

The model of aged-care funding adopted by Liberal–National Coalition parties since the John Howard government (1996–2007), and greatly extended since the Coalition's return to power in 2013, is privatisation overseen by the lightest of light-touch regulation and oversight. Under this model, owners and operators are incentivised to reduce costs and to pocket the difference between income and expenditure as profits. The greatest single expenditure in aged care is staffing and care. So, over time, the operators of private aged-care facilities reduced staffing costs by employing fewer people on lower wages. In effect, they replaced well-trained, permanent staff attached to one aged-care facility with gig workers paid at the lowest legal rates and employed at multiple sites.

When the pandemic hit, the low-paid gig-economy workers had very little capacity to do other than to keep working. The federal government had refused to extend JobKeeper to any such workers on contracts of less than twelve months. While operators benefited from a range of subsidies and tax breaks granted by the federal government in its March packages, they had no reason or incentive to vary the conditions of their workforce to provide stronger defences against coronavirus. The success of the first lockdown also swiftly reduced overall community transmission and therefore made it appear much less likely that workers shifting from one facility to the next would transmit the virus. The federal government and its agencies properly generated protocols and much useful information about infection control in aged care, as they did for healthcare workers. But they did so without understanding the impacts of the new reality created for many gig-economy workers by their economic packages. In aged care, the weaknesses in the structure of the industry were not remedied by aggressively stepping up compliance and supervision.

The problem with aged care in Victoria was foreshadowed by the impact of COVID-19 at Newmarch House in the Sydney suburb of Kingswood. The outbreak began on 11 April and lasted until 15 June. Some seventy-one residents and staff were infected, and seventeen residents succumbed to COVID-19. The event itself was handled as well as was possible, but an investigation into the outbreak revealed considerable problems with infection control, lack of PPE packs, staff shortages, poor training and an overall lack of clear communications.[19] The Newmarch House event should have prompted a searching review of the adequacy of measures taken across the aged-care sector and administered by the federal Department of Health. But once the infection crisis of March–May had passed, the attention of the federal government and its ministers waned. The Australian Government should have understood that the model of aged-care privatisation and labour hire was highly conducive to the spread of a virus in a pandemic. It could have remedied the most glaring weakness in the aged-care model by extending the JobKeeper provisions to all workers, and by ensuring that aged-care operators and owners abandoned the movement of workers from facility to facility, at least for the duration of the emergency.

The failure to implement the infection-control provisions of the *Emergency Response Plan* was reflected in the spread of infections that occurred among Victorian healthcare workers from the middle of May 2020 onwards. And as community infections increased over June and July, so did the risk that healthcare workers would be infected as they treated patients. It is clear that infection-control procedures were not implemented or applied effectively at many—though not all—hospitals and other healthcare facilities across the state. The spread of infection has also been attributed to the continuing shortages of PPE within hospitals and inconsistent guidelines for their use between different sites. This despite the ghastly examples of Italy and New York City receiving saturation coverage in the media only months before.

In Victoria, by the end of the second lockdown, over 3000 healthcare workers had been infected, mostly at their place of employment; almost 2000 residents of aged-care homes had been infected; and over 600 residents had died. These infections and deaths need not have happened. They could have been averted, as happened elsewhere in Australia and in New Zealand. This toll of illness, death, dislocation and misery was the result of poor political decisions. Politics propelled the Freedom Day campaign and undermined public support for sensible transition arrangements after the end of the first lockdown. It was a political decision by the federal government not to extend JobKeeper to all employees, thereby forcing gig-economy workers to keep working in ways that facilitated the spread of the virus. And academic stubbornness kept advisers committed to the flawed strategies outlined in the *Emergency Response Plan* in Victoria when these had been largely overtaken by developments.

By 2 June, the various jurisdictions of Australia and New Zealand had come as close to being COVID-free as was practically possible. This was because of the application of well-tested public health principles and policies. Nothing changed about the infectivity of coronavirus from March to June. It was really just another virus, able to be contained by simple precautionary measures. It is confounding, then, that the federal and Victorian governments, whose advisers were in constant contact, could evidently not manage the intersection of their various responsibilities so as to secure aged-care and healthcare facilities. There was very little understanding that the failure of the federal government's economic packages to provide financial support to low-paid and gig-economy workers set up perverse incentives that turbocharged the second wave. In this case, the deep fault lines in the outmoded structures of the Australian federation created confusion and were compounded by a lack of clarity and transparency at both the federal and Victorian levels.

All that was required to cement the achievements of the March–May lockdowns was the quiet, calm and methodical implementation of what had worked best to stop the spread of coronavirus. And, of course, this meant the abandonment of policies that had failed or fallen short. The virus could not thrive, indeed it could hardly survive, where these principles and policies were applied.

The only friend the virus has is politics.

PANDEMICS CREATE NEW POLITICS

Bad politics made Australia's coronavirus pandemic much harder to deal with than it ought to have been. It took about nine months from the first reported Australian case at the end of January 2020 until all Australian states and territories were united around the goal of zero local transmissions. In that time, some 27 000 people were infected and some 900 people had tragically died from COVID-19. Most of these infections and deaths were caused by the impact of an entirely predictable and avoidable second wave that struck in only one state: Victoria.

Poor strategic planning prepared behind a veil of secrecy and based on an inappropriate model created uncertainty during the critical months of February and March. In the confusion, the Australian Government took a series of economic decisions that ended twenty-nine years of uninterrupted economic growth, plunged the country into a deep recession, crippled many of the most productive sectors of the economy, and drove millions into underemployment and unemployment. The economic and social transformation caused by these rash and radical decisions will long impact the lives of Australians after the impacts of coronavirus itself have passed.

The repudiation on 22 March of Australia's preferred model for dealing with coronavirus meant that, at the very last possible moment, the nation veered away from the fate that engulfed the so-called peer countries of the United Kingdom and United States—those consulted by the Commonwealth Government's advisers. Rather, thanks to the common sense of the Australian people and the dedication of the hundreds of thousands who comprise the Australian public health sector, by the end of May, the country's coronavirus pandemic looked more like those of its Asian and Pacific neighbours than those of its British and American allies. By October 2020, the difference was even more remarkable, as evidenced by the statistics: Taiwan had experienced 510 cases and seven deaths, Vietnam 1074 cases and thirty-five deaths, Thailand 3523 cases and fifty-nine deaths, Singapore 57 000 cases and twenty-seven deaths, and New Zealand 1833 cases and twenty-five deaths, while the United Kingdom had endured 435 000 cases and 42 000 deaths, and the United States 7 140 000 cases and 205 000 deaths.

The Victorian and federal governments and their advisers did not use the breathing space afforded by the first lockdown to overhaul and remedy weaknesses in core functions and structures. Had they done so, the second wave would almost certainly never have crashed over Melbourne, and Australia's outcomes would have been that much better.

As the worst of the pandemic recedes, it is imperative that the entire response, the good and the bad, is scrutinised and assessed. The various reports commissioned into the *Ruby Princess*, Newmarch House and the Victorian hotel quarantine program examined significant events. But they were tightly defined and did not consider the bigger pictures of strategy, implementation and responsibility for outcomes.

Above all, it is time to reconstruct our health system around prevention. Only about 1–2 per cent of Australian health funding is allocated to prevention, while 98 per cent goes to care and treatment. We get what we pay for—care and treatment after the event— and don't get what we don't pay for—prevention of disease, illness and early deaths. In their response to HIV/AIDS and coronavirus, the Australian people showed they clearly grasp the wisdom of prevention. But the iron orthodoxy of the medical and scientific establishments prevails, to the detriment of public health and welfare.

In my opinion, these are the most pressing reforms that should be made if the Australian people are to be protected from the impacts of the inevitable next viral pandemic:

1   The *Biosecurity Act 2015* should be overhauled to remove all of the Commonwealth public health

functions from the national security structures and re-establish them in a new public health structure based in, or associated with, a revamped Department of Public Health.

2 Such a structure should be responsible for public health and disease prevention as well as the national coordination of pandemic planning and response. It must be grounded in default principles of transparency, accountability and open policymaking, and subject to oversight, scrutiny and review.

3 A comprehensive independent review of Australia's response to all aspects of the coronavirus pandemic is needed, including the interaction between health and economic policymaking.

4 All Australian governments must overhaul and upgrade their public health structures, funding and pandemic planning, drawing on the lessons and experience of the coronavirus pandemic, so as to ensure the primacy of prevention.

5 The WHO must be profoundly reformed so as to provide greater transparency, accountability and commitment to the prevention of pandemics.

6 Even with the return of the United States to WHO, member states, including Australia, will have to substantially increase WHO funding to implement the reform proposals that can be expected from the report of the Independent Panel for Pandemic Preparedness and Response.

7   There must be a root-and-branch overhaul of Australia's international relations, planning and liaison around pandemic planning, in particular to strengthen and deepen relations with peer countries in Asia and the Indo-Pacific.

No doubt a proper process of review and consultation with Australia's immensely well-credentialed public health professionals, and the public, would generate a template for much more effective global and national public health structures. But beyond practical reforms, we also have to understand that the coronavirus pandemic is just the most egregious symptom of the interlinked crisis that is overwhelming the planet. In 2020, the butcher's bill for decades of denying the science of both climate change and the threat of viral pandemics came due. In Australia, the year began with devastating fires caused by runaway emissions of carbon dioxide and other gases, followed immediately by the onset of a pandemic disease. Australia paid a heavy price for ignoring scientific truth.

Molecules of carbon dioxide and particles of coronavirus are simply expressions of the iron laws of physics, chemistry, biology and mathematics. It is delusional to believe that we can negotiate with molecules and viruses, or overcome their effects, by political means. The only way to prevail over the consequences of these iron laws of science is through the application of the same iron laws.

We know how to reduce emissions and decarbonise the atmosphere. We know how to eliminate coronavirus almost entirely by simple behavioural means and to finish the job with vaccines and treatments. We know how to prevent the next novel virus from morphing from a local problem into a global pandemic.

Bad politics is politics untethered from scientific truth. In 2020, bad politics crippled the health of millions, destroyed jobs and collapsed economies, all of it playing out as planetary heating accelerated. In 2021, only politics regrounded in scientific reality can begin to set the world on a path to the recovery of health, wealth and happiness.

POSTSCRIPT

In the wake of the Democrats' success in the November 2020 American election, the Biden administration is faced with the consequences of its predecessor's failure to manage coronavirus in the United States. From the outset, the Trump administration claimed that public health must be subordinated to politics, and so the stringent measures required to contain the virus were inconsistently applied. No effective border-control measures were imposed to stop the entry of infected travellers. The wearing of masks became submerged in the politics of the Trump re-election campaign.

The almost-unbelievable results of this rejection of science-based policies were three increasingly severe waves of coronavirus infection, the deaths of over 250 000 people, and economic carnage and dislocation on a scale unmatched since the Great Depression.

In the United States, the pandemic is now endemic.

President Biden must pursue strategies that combine sustained behavioural change, especially the universal use of masks, with improved therapeutics. The advent of vaccines will help, but vaccines are not cures. Their efficacy will only become apparent over months as more people are inoculated. This means that, as impossible as the politics of lockdowns might appear, they will have to be implemented if other efforts fail to bring the pandemic under control.

Of course, lockdowns can only be successful if sufficient funding is provided to underwrite the incomes of individuals and businesses. Money is the most potent vaccine of all. If the stimulus and support packages are inadequate, the containment measures will be largely ineffective.

Encouragingly, the Biden administration brings policies based on the best of American ingenuity, technology and expertise. Above all, President Biden's leadership is informed by science and evidence, not crude politics. The decision to rejoin the World Health Organization will restore American influence internationally and lead to far greater global cooperation and coordination around, for example, travel. But President Biden will also have to confront the uncomfortable social and economic truths exposed by this disaster.

The false dichotomy between the 'economy' and 'health' is at the heart of the neoliberal project that has held sway in capitalist nations since the 1980s. Spending on 'welfare' of all kinds, including public health and aged care, has been slashed as taxes on the wealthy have been slashed. But the foolishness of this approach has become apparent. The lack of spending on universal health provision, and above all prevention, was a driver of the US spread of coronavirus.

The redistribution of wealth from the rich to society generally strengthens public health care and limits the emergence of diseases—redistribution *is* prevention. Investment in robust prevention, detection and suppression measures would have stopped coronavirus before, not after, it became a pandemic. And the cost of these measures would have been a fraction of what has been spent to date. Neoliberal economics treats spending on prevention and public health as an expense, a drag on 'productivity', while the hundreds of billions thrown at vaccine research and production is welcomed as a boost to stock markets and profits.

Four decades ago, coincidentally at the time HIV/AIDS emerged, the Reagan administration embarked on a neoliberal experiment that subsequently swept the world. That experiment has run its course. It will now fall to a better, more decent American administration to learn the lessons of another viral pandemic, repudiate neoliberalism, and build back better.

ACKNOWLEDGEMENTS

For my parents, Bill and Inga.
And my family, Peter, Christine, Inga, Elliot and Ella.
And for Jose Antonio Costa dos Santos,
Sebastian Engelmann and Dr Li Wenliang.

~

My profound thanks to Louise Adler for suggesting that I write this book. I am very grateful to Paul Smitz for his accomplished editing, and to Greg Bain and the team at Monash University Publishing for bringing the project to fruition.

I am deeply grateful to my dear friends for their love, advice, support and encouragement, especially over the extraordinary year of 2020, and to those who reviewed the draft text, providing invaluable criticism, comments and suggestions that greatly improved the final text—for which I am solely responsible. Most are mentioned below, but some have wisely chosen to be held by me *in pectore*. I could not have written this without them.

Waheed Alli
John Black
James Bolster
Daniel Brace
Michael Cassel
Shawn Clackett
Aleks Dawson
Rob Finlayson
Mark Fittolani
Allan Gyngell
Wayne Harrison
Peter Hartcher
David Helms
David Henderson
Jennifer Hewett
Bilal Khalifeh
Nick Lucchinelli

Zann Maxwell
Wendy McCarthy
Les McDonald
Jeanine McMullan
Jenny Newton
Robert Newton
Steven Philpot
Julio Ribeiro
Heather Ridout
Marc Smith
Jonathan Stambolis
Norman Swan
John Watts
Tim West
Bill Whittaker
Brendon Williamson
Brendan Yeates

NOTES

1   Deborah Snow, 'Health Department Refuses to Release Minutes of Key COVID-19 Minutes', *The Sydney Morning Herald*, 6 September 2020.

2   The committee is to present its final report on or before 30 June 2022.

3   Thomas Friedman, in an article in *The New York Times* ('Is Trump Challenging Mother Nature to a Duel?', 19 May 2020), said that 'Mother Nature is just chemistry, biology and physics', to which I would add 'mathematics'.

4   See Richard J Hofstadter, *The Paranoid Style in American Politics*, Alfred A Knopf, New York, 1965.

5   Andrew Green, 'Obituary: Li Wenliang', *The Lancet*, vol. 395, no. 10 225, 29 February 2020, p. 682.

6   The Independent Panel for Pandemic Preparedness and Response, https://www.theindependentpanel.org (viewed October 2020).

7   Bob Woodward, *Rage*, Simon and Schuster, New York, 2020, p. xix.

8   Ibid., p. 286.

9   Ryan Goodman and Danielle Schulkin, 'Timeline of the Coronavirus Pandemic and U.S. Response', *Just Security*, 9 September 2020, http://www.justsecurity.org/69650/timeline-of-the-coronavirus-pandemic-and-u-s-response (viewed October 2020).

10   Jonathan Calvert, George Arbuthnott and Jonathan Leake, 'Coronavirus: 38 Days when Britain Sleepwalked into Disaster', *The Sunday Times*, 19 April 2020.

11   Michael Keane and Timothy Neal, 'Consumer Panic in the COVID-19 Pandemic', University of New South Wales & CEPAR, Sydney, 2020.

12   Stephen Grey and Andrew MacAskill, 'RPT Special Report: Johnson Listened to His Scientists about Coronavirus—But They Were Slow to Sound the Alarm', *Reuters*, 8 April 2020, p. 23; also see Jonathan Calvert, George Arbuthnott, Jonathan Leake and Dipesh Gadher, '22 Days of Dither and Delay on Coronavirus that Cost Thousands of British Lives', *The Sunday Times*, 23 May 2020.

13   Heather Stewart and Mattha Busby, 'Coronavirus: Science Chief Defends UK Plan from Criticism', *The Guardian*, 13 March 2020.

14   Imperial College COVID-19 Response Team, 'Report 9: Impact of Non-Pharmaceutical Interventions (NPIs) to Reduce COVID-19 Mortality and Healthcare Demand', Imperial College London, 16 March 2020.

15   Deborah Snow and Kate Aubusson, 'Shutting Down: How the Grim Reality of Coronavirus Hit Home', *The Sydney Morning Herald*, 7 September 2020.

16   Special Commission of Inquiry into the Ruby Princess, *Report*, NSW Government, Sydney, 14 August 2020.

17   Australian Institute of Health and Welfare, *Health Expenditure Australia 2017–18*, Health and Welfare Expenditure series, no. 65, 2019.

18   On 2 July 2020, the Victorian Governor in Council, on the recommendation of the Premier, appointed a board of inquiry, headed by the Honourable Jennifer Coate AO, to examine aspects of the COVID-19 Hotel Quarantine Program. At the time of writing, the COVID-19 Hotel Quarantine Inquiry was expected to report its findings in November 2020; see https://www.quarantineinquiry.vic.gov.au (viewed October 2020).

19   The Newmarch House COVID-19 Outbreak Independent Review was commissioned by the federal Department of Health to try and understand what happened. The review's *Final Report* was released on 20 August 2020; see https://www.health.gov.au/resources/publications/newmarch-house-covid-19-outbreak-independent-review (viewed October 2020).

IN THE NATIONAL INTEREST

Other books on the issues that matter: